# HEART DISEASE DIET COOKBOOK

Quick and Easy Low-Fat, Low-Sodium Recipes to Lower Blood Pressure, Reduce Cholesterol, and Promote Cardiovascular Health

**Beckham Brian**

Published by: [**Beckham Brian**], 2024.

# DISCLIAMER

The information provided in this book is intended for educational purposes only and is not a substitute for professional medical advice, diagnosis, or treatment. Always seek the advice of your physician or other qualified health provider with any questions you may have regarding a medical condition or dietary changes.

The recipes and dietary recommendations included in this book are based on research and the author's personal experience. However, individual needs may vary, and it is essential to consult with a healthcare professional before making significant changes to your diet, especially if you have existing health conditions or are taking medications.

The author and publisher of this book make no representations or warranties with respect to the accuracy, applicability, or completeness of the content. The recipes and information contained herein are provided "as is," without any guarantees or warranty of any kind. The author and publisher shall not be liable for any losses, injuries, or damages from the use of this information.

Furthermore, this book does not endorse any specific individual, product, website, organization, or other names referenced or mentioned within. All references are provided for informational purposes only. The author encourages readers to perform their own research and seek professional guidance before making decisions related to their health and nutrition.

By using this book, you agree to these terms and acknowledge that you are solely responsible for your dietary choices and health decisions.

# ABOUT THIS BOOK

The *Heart Disease Diet Cookbook* stands as a vital resource for anyone aiming to improve their cardiovascular health through diet. This cookbook is designed not only to provide delicious recipes but also to educate readers about the profound impact of nutrition on heart disease management. With an emphasis on low-fat and low-sodium meals, it empowers individuals to make informed dietary choices that can significantly lower blood pressure and reduce cholesterol levels. The book combines nutritional guidance with practical cooking advice, ensuring that heart-healthy eating becomes an achievable and enjoyable endeavor.

In addition to its comprehensive recipe collection, this cookbook offers invaluable insights into understanding heart disease and its implications. It lays the groundwork for recognizing the importance of a heart-healthy diet, demonstrating how essential nutrients contribute to overall cardiovascular wellness. The exploration of low-fat and low-sodium eating habits is particularly crucial, as it highlights the role these dietary adjustments play in combating heart-related ailments. By illustrating how to incorporate these principles into daily meals, the cookbook serves as a roadmap for lasting dietary changes that promote heart health.

Success stories within the book serve as a testament to the positive outcomes that can result from adhering to the dietary recommendations. These personal accounts inspire and motivate readers, demonstrating that it is indeed possible to achieve a healthier lifestyle with commitment and the right tools. Furthermore, the book provides practical tips for successful dietary changes, helping individuals navigate the challenges of adopting new eating habits while remaining motivated and focused on their health goals.

The cookbook also emphasizes the importance of meal planning and preparation, equipping readers with strategies for creating balanced grocery lists and preparing meals in advance. This approach is vital for maintaining consistency and ensuring that heart-healthy options are readily available. Understanding labels and ingredients is another critical aspect covered, guiding readers to identify hidden sources of sodium and unhealthy fats while selecting heart-healthy alternatives. By demystifying nutrition labels and ingredient lists, the book empowers readers to make better choices while shopping.

Moreover, the inclusion of special dietary needs, such as options for managing diabetes alongside heart disease or adapting recipes for gluten-free or vegan diets, broadens its appeal to a diverse audience. This cookbook recognizes that health journeys are not one-size-fits-all, providing tailored solutions for various lifestyles and dietary preferences. It also integrates exercise recommendations, underscoring the synergy between diet and physical activity in promoting heart health.

Ultimately, the *Heart Disease Diet Cookbook* is more than just a collection of recipes; it is a holistic guide to achieving and maintaining heart health. By merging practical cooking techniques with in-depth nutritional knowledge and personal success stories, it inspires readers to embrace a heart-healthy lifestyle that is both sustainable and enjoyable. This resource stands as a beacon of hope and guidance for individuals seeking to take control of their heart health through informed dietary choices.

# Table of Contents

# The Importance of This Diet Cookbook

Heart disease is a leading health issue globally, making dietary changes crucial for managing and preventing cardiovascular conditions. This cookbook is specifically designed to address the need for a heart-healthy diet by offering quick and easy low-fat, low-sodium recipes. By focusing on reducing fat and sodium intake, the recipes in this book help lower blood pressure and cholesterol levels, which are essential for maintaining cardiovascular health.

Each recipe is crafted to simplify the process of cooking heart-healthy meals without compromising on flavor. The cookbook ensures that even those with busy schedules can prepare nutritious dishes that support a heart-healthy lifestyle. By following these recipes, readers can make informed food choices that contribute to long-term cardiovascular wellness.

# How This Book Can Help You Achieve a Better Life

This cookbook provides practical guidance for individuals looking to improve their heart health through diet. The easy-to-follow recipes are designed to fit seamlessly into daily routines, making it manageable for beginners to stick to a heart-healthy eating plan. The focus on low-fat and low-sodium ingredients means that readers can enjoy delicious meals while making significant strides in lowering their blood pressure and cholesterol.

Additionally, the book includes tips and strategies for making heart-healthy cooking a habit, such as meal prep ideas and ingredient substitutions. By integrating these recipes into your diet, you not only enhance your cardiovascular health but also develop healthier eating habits that can lead to an overall better quality of life.

# Success Stories

## 1. Mary Johnson

**Background:** Mary, a 55-year-old schoolteacher, had been struggling with high blood pressure and elevated cholesterol for years. Despite trying various medications, she found it challenging to maintain a heart-healthy diet.

**Approach:** Mary discovered the "Heart Disease Diet Cookbook" through a friend's recommendation and decided to give it a try. She began by incorporating a few recipes from the book into her weekly meal plan, focusing on the low-fat and low-sodium options.

**Results:** Within three months, Mary noticed a significant drop in her blood pressure and cholesterol levels. Her doctor was impressed with the progress and encouraged her to continue with the diet. Mary reported feeling more energetic and less dependent on her medication, which was a major victory for her.

## 2. David Ramirez

**Background:** David, a 62-year-old retired firefighter, had a history of heart disease in his family. Despite regular exercise, his cholesterol levels remained high, and he struggled with maintaining a heart-healthy diet.

**Approach:** After a particularly concerning check-up, David decided to take a proactive approach by adopting the diet outlined in the "Heart Disease Diet Cookbook." He meticulously followed the recipes and incorporated them into his daily routine, focusing on portion control and balanced meals.

**Results:** By the end of the year, David experienced a remarkable reduction in his cholesterol levels and improved heart function. His cardiologist was thrilled with the results and praised the cookbook for its practical and effective approach. David felt a renewed sense of control over his health and credited the book for his positive changes.

### 3. Lisa Thompson

**Background:** Lisa, a 48-year-old marketing executive, had recently been diagnosed with prehypertension and was advised to make dietary changes to prevent further health issues. She was overwhelmed by conflicting dietary advice and sought a straightforward solution.

**Approach:** Lisa came across the "Heart Disease Diet Cookbook" while researching heart-healthy diets online. She was drawn to the book's focus on easy-to-prepare recipes that fit her busy schedule. She committed to following the cookbook's guidelines and began meal prepping on weekends.

**Results:** Within six months, Lisa saw a significant improvement in her blood pressure and overall cardiovascular health. Her doctor was impressed by the effectiveness of the diet and noted that Lisa had successfully avoided the need for medication. Lisa felt more confident in her ability to manage her health and praised the cookbook for its simplicity and effectiveness.

## 4. John and Karen Lee

**Background:** John and Karen, a married couple in their early 60s, both faced high cholesterol and high blood pressure. They wanted to make a joint effort to improve their health but struggled to find a diet plan that suited both their tastes and preferences.

**Approach:** They decided to try the "Heart Disease Diet Cookbook" together, as the book offered a variety of recipes that could cater to both their needs. They enjoyed experimenting with different meals and found the recipes to be both enjoyable and easy to prepare.

**Results:** Over the course of a year, John and Karen both experienced significant improvements in their cholesterol levels and blood pressure. Their joint commitment to the diet brought them closer together and made meal planning a fun and collaborative experience. Their success story was featured in a local health magazine, showcasing the cookbook's impact on their lives.

# Introduction

## <u>Understanding Heart Disease and Its Impact</u>

Heart disease, or cardiovascular disease, encompasses a range of conditions affecting the heart and blood vessels, including coronary artery disease, heart attacks, and hypertension. It often results from factors like high blood pressure, high cholesterol, and a sedentary lifestyle. These conditions can lead to the narrowing of arteries, reducing blood flow and increasing the risk of heart attacks and strokes. Understanding these risks helps in managing and preventing heart disease through lifestyle changes.

The impact of heart disease extends beyond physical health, affecting quality of life and increasing healthcare costs. Individuals with heart disease may experience symptoms like chest pain, fatigue, and shortness of breath. Early intervention and lifestyle modifications, including dietary changes, are crucial for managing symptoms and reducing long-term risks associated with heart disease.

## The Importance of a Heart-Healthy Diet

A heart-healthy diet plays a critical role in managing and preventing heart disease. It emphasizes foods that reduce inflammation, lower cholesterol, and maintain healthy blood pressure levels. Key components include high-fiber foods like fruits, vegetables, whole grains, and lean proteins. These foods help in reducing cholesterol levels and improving overall cardiovascular health.

By adopting a heart-healthy diet, you can significantly lower your risk of heart disease. Reducing the intake of saturated fats, trans fats, and high-sodium foods helps prevent arterial plaque buildup and maintains healthy blood pressure. A balanced diet not only supports heart health but also enhances overall well-being and energy levels.

# Overview of Low-Fat and Low-Sodium Eating

Low-fat and low-sodium eating focuses on reducing the intake of fats and sodium to improve heart health. Low-fat diets help lower cholesterol levels while reducing sodium intake prevents fluid retention and high blood pressure. Opt for lean proteins such as chicken breast, fish, and legumes, and choose cooking methods like grilling or steaming over frying.

To implement a low-sodium diet, use herbs and spices to flavor foods instead of salt. Incorporate fresh, whole foods and avoid processed items that often contain hidden sodium. Understanding food labels and choosing products with reduced fat and sodium can simplify dietary adjustments and contribute to better cardiovascular health.

# How This Cookbook Will Help You

This cookbook is designed to simplify heart-healthy eating with quick and easy low-fat, low-sodium recipes. Each recipe is crafted to support cardiovascular health while being delicious and easy to prepare. The cookbook provides clear instructions and ingredient lists that focus on heart-friendly foods, making it straightforward to incorporate healthy meals into your daily routine.

By following the recipes, you can enjoy a variety of meals that adhere to dietary guidelines for heart health. The cookbook includes practical tips and substitutions to help you maintain a balanced diet, making it easier to stick to dietary changes and improve your overall cardiovascular well-being.

# Tips for Successful Dietary Changes

Successful dietary changes involve gradual adjustments and consistent habits. Start by setting realistic goals, such as incorporating one new heart-healthy meal per week. Track your progress and make adjustments as needed to stay on course. It's also helpful to plan meals ahead and prepare healthy snacks to avoid reaching for unhealthy options.

Engaging in meal planning and cooking can make dietary changes more manageable. Involve family members in your journey by preparing meals together and exploring new recipes. Educating yourself about nutrition and understanding food labels will empower you to make informed choices, ensuring a smoother transition to a heart-healthy lifestyle.

# CHAPTER 1

## <u>What a Healthy Diet Must Include</u>

### Essential Nutrients for Heart Health

To maintain heart health, focus on incorporating key nutrients into your diet. Essential vitamins and minerals like potassium, magnesium, and vitamins C and E help regulate blood pressure and reduce oxidative stress. Foods rich in these nutrients include leafy greens, bananas, and citrus fruits. Additionally, omega-3 fatty acids from sources like flaxseeds, walnuts, and fatty fish support heart function by reducing inflammation and lowering triglyceride levels.

Incorporate these nutrients into daily meals by adding spinach or kale to smoothies, snacking on nuts, and including fish like salmon in your weekly meal plan. This approach ensures that you're consistently providing your body with the necessary elements to support cardiovascular health.

# Importance of Fiber and Whole Grains

Fiber is crucial for heart health as it helps lower cholesterol levels and improves digestion. Whole grains, such as oats, brown rice, and quinoa, are excellent sources of soluble fiber, which binds to cholesterol and helps remove it from the body. Aim to include whole grains in every meal to reap their cardiovascular benefits.

Start your day with a bowl of oatmeal or add quinoa to salads and soups. Substituting refined grains with whole grains in recipes ensures that you're getting enough fiber to support heart health. This simple dietary change can significantly impact your cholesterol levels and overall cardiovascular well-being.

# Role of Healthy Fats and Protein

Healthy fats, such as those found in avocados, nuts, and olive oil, are essential for heart health. They help reduce LDL cholesterol levels and provide anti-inflammatory benefits. Include these fats in your diet while avoiding trans fats and saturated fats found in fried foods and processed snacks. Lean proteins from sources like chicken breast, tofu, and legumes support muscle health and overall cardiovascular function.

Prepare meals using olive oil for cooking or add avocado slices to salads. Choose lean protein options for main dishes to balance your fat intake while maintaining heart health. This approach helps ensure you're getting the right kinds of fats and proteins for a heart-healthy diet.

# Recommended Daily Values and Portion Sizes

Understanding recommended daily values (RDVs) helps you make informed dietary choices. For heart health, aim for less than 2,300 mg of sodium per day and limit saturated fat to less than 10% of total daily calories. Portion sizes are crucial; for example, a serving of protein should be about the size of a deck of cards, and whole grains should fill about a quarter of your plate.

Use measuring cups and a food scale to control portion sizes, and read nutrition labels to keep track of sodium and fat intake. By adhering to these guidelines, you can better manage your diet and support cardiovascular health effectively.

# Balancing Macronutrients for Optimal Health

Balancing macronutrients—carbohydrates, proteins, and fats—is key to a heart-healthy diet. Aim for a balance where about 50% of your daily calories come from carbohydrates, 20-25% from proteins, and 25-30% from fats. Opt for complex carbohydrates like whole grains, lean proteins, and healthy fats to support cardiovascular health.

Plan meals to include a mix of these macronutrients: for example, pair a whole grain like quinoa with lean chicken and a side of vegetables sautéed in olive oil. This balanced approach helps ensure that your body gets the nutrients it needs to maintain heart health and overall well-being.

# CHAPTER 2

## Best Grocery Store Foods to Stockpile

### Heart-Healthy Vegetables and Fruits

Incorporate a variety of colorful vegetables and fruits into your diet to boost heart health. Focus on leafy greens like spinach and kale, which are rich in vitamins and antioxidants. Fruits such as berries, apples, and oranges offer essential nutrients and fiber that help lower cholesterol levels. Aim for at least five servings of vegetables and fruits daily. For practical use, add a handful of spinach to your morning smoothie or top your cereal with fresh berries.

To make it easy, plan meals around these ingredients. For example, prepare a hearty vegetable soup with carrots, tomatoes, and bell peppers, or enjoy a mixed fruit salad as a refreshing snack. Use these fruits and vegetables in place of processed snacks and dishes to naturally reduce sodium and unhealthy fats in your diet.

## Whole Grains and Legumes

Whole grains and legumes are crucial for heart health due to their high fiber content, which helps lower cholesterol and regulate blood pressure. Opt for brown rice, quinoa, and whole wheat bread over refined grains. Legumes like beans, lentils, and chickpeas are excellent sources of plant-based protein and fiber. Incorporate these into your diet by using them as a base for salads, soups, or side dishes.

Cook a large batch of quinoa or brown rice and use it throughout the week in different meals. For instance, make a hearty bean chili or a lentil salad. These grains and legumes are not only nutritious but also versatile, making it easy to integrate them into various recipes without extensive preparation.

## Lean Proteins and Healthy Fats

Choose lean proteins such as chicken breast, turkey, and fish, which provide essential amino acids without excessive saturated fats. Opt for cooking methods like grilling, baking, or steaming instead of frying. Include healthy fats from sources like avocados, nuts, and olive oil, which support cardiovascular health. For a practical approach, prepare grilled chicken with a side of roasted vegetables drizzled with olive oil.

Incorporate these proteins and fats into balanced meals. For example, enjoy a grilled salmon fillet with a side of quinoa and steamed broccoli. Snack on a handful of almonds or a slice of avocado on whole-grain toast to boost your intake of healthy fats and keep your heart in good shape.

# Low-Sodium and Low-Fat Dairy Options

Select dairy products that are low in sodium and fat to reduce your risk of heart disease. Options include skim or 1% milk, low-fat yogurt, and reduced-fat cheese. These alternatives provide the necessary calcium and protein without the added saturated fats and sodium found in full-fat versions. Substitute these products in recipes where cream or full-fat dairy is typically used.

For practical use, start your day with a serving of low-fat yogurt topped with fruit or add a splash of skim milk to your morning coffee. Choose reduced-fat cheese for sandwiches or salads to maintain flavor while lowering fat intake. These swaps are simple yet effective in managing heart health.

# Staples for Quick and Easy Meals

Stock your kitchen with heart-healthy staples that facilitate quick meal preparation. Essentials include canned beans, whole-grain pasta, frozen vegetables, and low-sodium broth. These items can be used to create nutritious meals in a matter of minutes. For instance, use canned beans to make a quick chili or add frozen vegetables to a stir-fry with whole-grain pasta.

Prepare meal components in advance, like chopping vegetables or cooking grains, to streamline your cooking process. This approach not only saves time but also ensures you have ready-to-use ingredients that align with a heart-healthy diet. By having these staples on hand, you can easily whip up meals that support cardiovascular health without the need for complex recipes.

# CHAPTER 3

# <u>Appetizers</u>

## Fresh Vegetable Platter with Low-Fat Dips

To create a fresh vegetable platter, select a variety of colorful vegetables such as bell peppers, carrots, cucumbers, and cherry tomatoes. Wash and cut the vegetables into bite-sized pieces, arranging them on a platter for a visually appealing presentation.

For the low-fat dips, prepare options like a yogurt-based herb dip or a tangy salsa. Mix Greek yogurt with chopped fresh herbs such as dill and chives, adding a squeeze of lemon juice for extra flavor. Alternatively, blend tomatoes, onions, cilantro, and lime juice to make a simple salsa that pairs well with crunchy veggies.

Serve the platter as an appetizer or a healthy snack. The vegetables provide essential nutrients, while the low-fat dips add flavor without excess calories. Ensure the dips are served in separate bowls to prevent mixing and to maintain freshness. This approach helps keep the meal light and heart-healthy, making it easy to stick to a diet that supports cardiovascular health.

## Baked Sweet Potato Fries

Baked sweet potato fries are a heart-healthy alternative to traditional fries. Begin by peeling and cutting sweet potatoes into thin strips. Toss the strips in a mixture of olive oil, paprika, garlic powder, and a pinch of salt. Spread them evenly on a baking sheet lined with parchment paper to avoid sticking. Bake in a preheated oven at 425°F (220°C) for 20-25 minutes, flipping halfway through for even cooking. The result is crispy, golden fries with less fat compared to deep-fried options.

These fries are rich in vitamins and antioxidants, making them a nutritious choice for anyone looking to reduce cholesterol and manage blood pressure. Serve them as a side dish or a snack, paired with a low-fat dipping sauce if desired. By baking instead of frying, you cut down on unhealthy fats while enjoying a tasty treat that supports heart health.

## Stuffed Mushrooms with Spinach

For stuffed mushrooms, start by removing the stems from large mushroom caps and setting them aside. Sauté finely chopped mushroom stems with garlic and onions in a small amount of olive oil until soft. Add chopped fresh spinach to the pan and cook until wilted. Combine this mixture with whole wheat breadcrumbs and a sprinkle of Parmesan cheese. Spoon the filling into the mushroom caps and place them on a baking sheet. Bake at 375°F (190°C) for 15-20 minutes, or until the mushrooms are tender and the tops are golden.

These stuffed mushrooms make a delicious and heart-healthy appetizer or side dish. The spinach provides essential vitamins and minerals, while the mushrooms offer fiber and antioxidants. By using whole wheat breadcrumbs and limiting cheese, you keep the dish low in fat and sodium, aligning it with dietary guidelines for heart health.

## Cucumber and Avocado Bites

To prepare cucumber and avocado bites, slice cucumbers into thick rounds and hollow out the centers slightly to create a small well. Mash ripe avocados with a squeeze of lime juice, a pinch of salt, and a dash of black pepper. Spoon the avocado mixture into the cucumber wells, garnishing with a sprinkle of chopped cilantro or a small piece of cherry tomato. Arrange the bites on a serving plate for a refreshing and visually appealing appetizer.

These bites are low in sodium and fat while offering healthy fats from the avocado. They are easy to prepare and serve as a light, heart-healthy snack.

The cucumber adds crunch and hydration, while the avocado provides beneficial nutrients like potassium and monounsaturated fats, supporting overall cardiovascular health.

## Tomato and Basil Bruschetta

For tomato and basil bruschetta, start by toasting slices of whole-grain baguette or crusty bread until crisp. Dice ripe tomatoes and mix them with finely chopped fresh basil, a drizzle of olive oil, and a splash of balsamic vinegar. Season the mixture with a pinch of salt and pepper to taste. Spoon the tomato mixture onto the toasted bread slices just before serving to prevent sogginess.

This bruschetta is a flavorful and heart-healthy appetizer. The tomatoes provide antioxidants and vitamins, while the basil adds a burst of freshness. Using whole-grain bread and limiting olive oil ensures the recipe remains low in fat and sodium, making it suitable for those managing blood pressure and cholesterol levels.

# CHAPTER 4

# <u>Breakfast</u>

## Oatmeal with Fresh Berries and Nuts

To prepare oatmeal with fresh berries and nuts, start by cooking rolled oats according to package instructions, typically simmering in water or low-fat milk for about 5 minutes. Once the oats are soft and creamy, stir in a handful of fresh berries, such as blueberries or strawberries, for natural sweetness and a burst of flavor. Top with a sprinkle of chopped nuts like almonds or walnuts to add a crunchy texture and heart-healthy fats.

For an extra nutritional boost, consider adding a dash of cinnamon or a small spoonful of flaxseeds. This not only enhances the flavor but also provides additional fiber and omega-3 fatty acids, which are beneficial for heart health. Serve immediately to enjoy a warm, satisfying breakfast that supports cardiovascular well-being.

## Greek Yogurt Parfait with Honey and Granola

Creating a Greek yogurt parfait is a simple way to enjoy a heart-healthy snack. Begin by layering Greek yogurt, which is high in protein and low in fat, in a bowl or glass. Add a drizzle of honey for natural sweetness and a layer of granola for a satisfying crunch. The combination of yogurt and granola provides a balanced mix of protein, fiber, and healthy fats, promoting heart health and keeping you full.

To further enhance the parfait, mix in some fresh fruit such as sliced bananas or berries. This adds vitamins, antioxidants, and additional fiber, all of which contribute to overall cardiovascular health. Assemble and enjoy as a quick breakfast or snack that supports a low-fat, low-sodium diet.

# Whole Grain Avocado Toast

Making whole-grain avocado toast is straightforward and nutritious. Toast a slice of whole-grain bread until it's crispy. While the bread is toasting, mash a ripe avocado with a fork, adding a pinch of salt and pepper for flavor. Spread the mashed avocado evenly over the toasted bread, and for extra heart-healthy benefits, top with a sprinkle of chia seeds or a few slices of cherry tomatoes.

For additional flavor and nutrition, consider adding a drizzle of olive oil or a squeeze of lemon juice. These ingredients not only enhance the taste but also provide healthy fats and antioxidants. This simple meal is an excellent choice for anyone looking to maintain a low-sodium, low-fat diet while promoting cardiovascular health.

## Egg White and Vegetable Omelet

To prepare an egg white and vegetable omelet, start by whisking egg whites in a bowl until they are slightly frothy. Heat a non-stick skillet over medium heat and pour in the egg whites, allowing them to cook until they start to set. Add chopped vegetables such as spinach, bell peppers, and onions to one-half of the omelet, cooking until the vegetables are tender.

Fold the omelet in half and cook for an additional minute to ensure it is fully set. This dish is rich in protein and low in fat, making it an ideal choice for a heart-healthy diet. Serve immediately for a satisfying breakfast or lunch that helps lower cholesterol and blood pressure.

## Smoothie with Spinach and Fruit

Preparing a smoothie with spinach and fruit is both quick and nutritious. Start by blending a handful of fresh spinach with a cup of your favorite fruit, such as bananas, berries, or mangoes. Add a cup of low-fat yogurt or a splash of almond milk to achieve a creamy texture and boost protein content.

For added heart health benefits, include a tablespoon of chia seeds or flaxseeds, which are rich in omega-3 fatty acids. Blend until smooth and enjoy a refreshing, nutrient-packed smoothie that supports cardiovascular health while keeping your sodium and fat intake low.

# CHAPTER 5

# <u>Lunch</u>

## Grilled Chicken Salad with Lemon Vinaigrette

For a heart-healthy grilled chicken salad, start by marinating chicken breasts in a mix of lemon juice, garlic, and a touch of olive oil for flavor without added fat. Grill the chicken over medium heat for about 6-8 minutes per side, or until fully cooked and juices run clear. Once cooled, slice the chicken into strips and toss it with mixed greens, cherry tomatoes, cucumber, and red onion.

To make the lemon vinaigrette, whisk together fresh lemon juice, a teaspoon of Dijon mustard, a tablespoon of olive oil, and a pinch of salt and pepper. Drizzle the dressing over the salad just before serving. This simple preparation is not only low in sodium but also helps maintain optimal blood pressure and cholesterol levels.

## Quinoa and Black Bean Salad

Cook quinoa according to package instructions, usually simmering it in water for about 15 minutes until fluffy. Allow it to cool before mixing with cooked black beans, diced red bell peppers, corn, and chopped cilantro. This combination provides a high-protein, fiber-rich base that aids in lowering cholesterol and supporting heart health.

For the dressing, combine lime juice, a touch of olive oil, minced garlic, and a pinch of cumin. Toss the quinoa mixture with the dressing and let it sit for at least 30 minutes to allow the flavors to meld. This salad is a versatile, low-fat option that can be served as a main dish or a side.

## Turkey and Veggie Wraps

To prepare these wraps, start by cooking ground turkey in a skillet with a splash of olive oil, seasoned with paprika, garlic powder, and black pepper. Sauté diced vegetables such as bell peppers, zucchini, and onions until tender. Combine the turkey with the veggies for a flavorful filling.

Use whole-grain or low-sodium wraps and fill them with the turkey and veggie mixture. Add a handful of spinach or arugula for extra nutrients. Roll up tightly and slice in half. These wraps provide a satisfying, low-sodium meal that's easy to prepare and helps with maintaining heart health.

## Lentil Soup with Fresh Herbs

Begin by sautéing onions, garlic, and carrots in a pot with a small amount of olive oil until softened. Add rinsed lentils, diced tomatoes, and low-sodium vegetable broth. Simmer the soup for about 30 minutes or until the lentils are tender. Stir in chopped fresh herbs like parsley or thyme for added flavor.

For extra flavor, season with a pinch of cumin and black pepper. This soup is rich in fiber and plant-based protein, making it excellent for heart health. Serve hot with a side of whole-grain bread for a complete, heart-healthy meal.

# Sweet Potato and Chickpea Bowl

Roast diced sweet potatoes and canned chickpeas on a baking sheet with a drizzle of olive oil and a sprinkle of smoked paprika at 400°F for 25-30 minutes or until crispy. In a bowl, combine the roasted sweet potatoes and chickpeas with a mix of greens such as kale or spinach.

Top with a dollop of plain Greek yogurt mixed with lemon juice and a pinch of cumin. This bowl provides a balance of complex carbs, protein, and healthy fats, which supports cardiovascular health and keeps sodium levels low. Enjoy this dish warm or cold as a nutritious and filling meal.

# CHAPTER 6

# <u>Dinner</u>

## Baked Salmon with Lemon and Dill

For a heart-healthy meal, start by preheating your oven to 375°F (190°C). Place salmon fillets on a baking sheet lined with parchment paper. Season each fillet with a sprinkle of salt and pepper, then top with thin slices of lemon and fresh dill. Bake for 15-20 minutes or until the salmon flakes easily with a fork. This simple preparation ensures you get a flavorful, low-fat, and heart-healthy meal that supports cardiovascular health.

To enhance the flavor without adding extra sodium, you can also squeeze a bit of fresh lemon juice over the fillets before serving. Pair this dish with a side of steamed vegetables or a mixed greens salad for a complete, heart-friendly meal.

## Stuffed Bell Peppers with Brown Rice

Begin by preheating your oven to 375°F (190°C). Cut the tops off bell peppers and remove the seeds. In a skillet, cook chopped onions, garlic, and any desired vegetables until tender. Stir in cooked brown rice, a can of diced tomatoes, and your favorite herbs and spices. Stuff the mixture into the bell peppers, place them upright in a baking dish and bake for 30-35 minutes. This dish is low in fat and sodium, making it a nutritious option for heart health.

For added protein, you can mix in some lean ground turkey or chicken into the rice filling. This not only boosts the nutritional value but also makes the dish more filling and satisfying.

# Spaghetti Squash with Tomato Basil Sauce

To prepare spaghetti squash, cut it in half lengthwise and remove the seeds. Place the halves cut-side down on a baking sheet and bake at 400°F (200°C) for about 40 minutes, or until tender. Once cooked, use a fork to scrape out the strands of squash. For the sauce, heat olive oil in a pan, add minced garlic and cook until fragrant. Add canned crushed tomatoes and fresh basil, simmer for 10 minutes, and then pour over the cooked squash. This meal provides a low-carb alternative to traditional pasta while still delivering a rich, satisfying flavor.

For a richer sauce, consider adding a splash of low-sodium vegetable broth or a pinch of red pepper flakes for a bit of heat. The spaghetti squash serves as a great base for the tangy and herbaceous tomato sauce, making it a great option for lowering blood pressure and cholesterol.

# Grilled Portobello Mushrooms

Start by cleaning Portobello mushrooms and removing the stems. Brush each cap with a mixture of olive oil, balsamic vinegar, garlic, and a pinch of salt and pepper. Heat a grill or grill pan over medium-high heat and place the mushroom caps on it. Grill for about 5-7 minutes on each side, or until tender and nicely charred. This method preserves the mushrooms' natural flavors and provides a satisfying, low-fat option that supports heart health.

For extra flavor, consider marinating the mushrooms in the oil mixture for a few hours before grilling. Serve them as a main dish or sliced on top of a salad for a hearty, plant-based meal that contributes to cardiovascular wellness.

# Chicken Stir-Fry with Vegetables

To make this heart-healthy stir-fry, start by cutting boneless, skinless chicken breast into thin strips. Heat a small amount of olive oil in a large skillet or wok over medium-high heat. Add the chicken and cook until browned and cooked through. Remove the chicken and add a variety of vegetables like bell peppers, broccoli, and carrots to the skillet. Stir-fry until tender-crisp. Return the chicken to the pan and add a low-sodium soy sauce or a splash of low-sodium chicken broth. Cook for a few more minutes and serve over brown rice or quinoa.

To enhance the flavor without adding extra sodium, you can use fresh ginger and garlic in the stir-fry. This dish provides a balanced mix of protein and vegetables while keeping the fat and sodium content low, promoting overall cardiovascular health.

# CHAPTER 7

# Desserts

## Baked Apples with Cinnamon

To prepare Baked Apples with Cinnamon, first, preheat your oven to 350°F (175°C). Core and peel 4 medium-sized apples, then place them in a baking dish. In a small bowl, mix 2 tablespoons of cinnamon with 1 tablespoon of honey or a low-calorie sweetener, then spoon this mixture into the hollowed centers of the apples. Bake for about 25 minutes or until the apples are tender. For extra flavor, you can add a sprinkle of nutmeg or a few chopped walnuts on top before baking.

This dish is not only heart-healthy but also easy to prepare. The natural sweetness of the apples combined with the warm cinnamon creates a comforting dessert that is low in fat and sodium. It provides a satisfying end to any meal without compromising your dietary goals.

# Chia Seed Pudding with Fresh Fruit

To make Chia Seed Pudding with Fresh Fruit, start by mixing 3 tablespoons of chia seeds with 1 cup of unsweetened almond milk or any low-fat milk alternative. Stir in a teaspoon of vanilla extract and let the mixture sit in the refrigerator for at least 4 hours or overnight to allow the chia seeds to absorb the liquid and form a pudding-like texture. Once set, top the pudding with a handful of fresh berries or sliced fruit of your choice.

Chia seeds are a great source of omega-3 fatty acids and fiber, which are beneficial for heart health. This pudding is simple to prepare and can be customized with different fruits and flavors, making it a versatile and nutritious option for breakfast or a snack.

# Low-Fat Berry Sorbet

To create Low-Fat Berry Sorbet, blend 2 cups of mixed berries (such as strawberries, blueberries, and raspberries) with 1/2 cup of water and 2 tablespoons of honey or a low-calorie sweetener in a food processor until smooth. Pour the mixture into a shallow dish and freeze for about 2 hours, stirring every 30 minutes to break up ice crystals. Once the sorbet is firm but still scoopable, serve immediately for a refreshing, low-fat treat.

Berry sorbet is a delicious way to enjoy fruit without added fats or high sodium. The natural sweetness of the berries, combined with the cooling effect of the sorbet, makes it a perfect dessert for hot days while supporting cardiovascular health.

# Whole Wheat Banana Bread

For Whole Wheat Banana Bread, preheat your oven to 350°F (175°C). In a mixing bowl, combine 1 1/2 cups of whole wheat flour with 1 teaspoon of baking powder and 1/2 teaspoon of baking soda. In another bowl, mash 3 ripe bananas and mix in 1/4 cup of unsweetened applesauce and 1/2 cup of honey or a low-calorie sweetener. Combine the wet and dry ingredients, then pour the batter into a greased loaf pan. Bake for 50-60 minutes or until a toothpick inserted in the center comes out clean.

This banana bread is a heart-healthy alternative to traditional recipes, offering the benefits of whole wheat flour and reduced fat. It's an excellent choice for breakfast or a snack, providing a good source of dietary fiber and potassium from the bananas.

## Fruit Salad with Citrus Dressing

To make a Fruit Salad with Citrus Dressing, chop a variety of fresh fruits such as apples, oranges, grapes, and kiwi into bite-sized pieces and mix them in a large bowl. For the dressing, whisk together 2 tablespoons of fresh lemon juice, 1 tablespoon of honey or a low-calorie sweetener, and a pinch of finely grated lime zest. Drizzle the dressing over the fruit salad and toss gently to combine.

This fruit salad is vibrant and packed with vitamins, making it a heart-healthy option. The citrus dressing adds a zesty flavor without extra fat or sodium, enhancing the natural sweetness of the fruits and making it a refreshing addition to any meal.

# CHAPTER 8

# Vegetarian Recipes

## Spicy Black Bean and Corn Tacos

These tacos are a heart-healthy choice, packed with fiber and low in fat. Start by heating a skillet over medium heat and add a tablespoon of olive oil. Sauté chopped onions and garlic until translucent, then stir in canned black beans, drained and rinsed, along with fresh or frozen corn kernels. Season with cumin, chili powder, and a pinch of cayenne pepper to taste. Cook for 5-7 minutes, allowing the flavors to meld.

To assemble, warm whole-grain tortillas and fill them with the black bean and corn mixture. Top with shredded lettuce, diced tomatoes, and a squeeze of lime juice for extra freshness. Garnish with chopped cilantro if desired. This recipe is simple to prepare and offers a satisfying meal with reduced sodium and no added fats.

## Vegetable and Tofu Stir-Fry

This quick stir-fry provides a nutritious and flavorful way to enjoy a variety of vegetables. Begin by pressing and cubing firm tofu, then sauté it in a non-stick pan with a splash of low-sodium soy sauce until golden brown. Remove the tofu and set aside. In the same pan, add a mix of vegetables such as bell peppers, broccoli, and snap peas. Stir-fry until tender-crisp, about 5 minutes.

Return the tofu to the pan and add a sauce made from a tablespoon of low-sodium soy sauce, a teaspoon of grated ginger, and a tablespoon of rice vinegar. Stir well to combine and heat through. Serve over brown rice or quinoa for a complete meal. This dish is low in fat and sodium while rich in protein and fiber.

# Lentil and Vegetable Curry

This hearty curry is perfect for a low-fat, heart-healthy meal. Start by sautéing chopped onions, garlic, and ginger in a pot with a bit of olive oil. Add a mixture of spices like turmeric, cumin, and coriander. Stir in dried lentils, diced tomatoes, and vegetable broth. Simmer until the lentils are tender, about 20 minutes.

In the last 10 minutes of cooking, add chopped vegetables such as carrots, bell peppers, and spinach. Adjust seasoning with salt and pepper to taste. Serve the curry over a bed of whole-grain rice or alongside a piece of whole-grain naan for a complete and satisfying meal.

# Spinach and Mushroom Stuffed Peppers

These stuffed peppers are both flavorful and nutritious. Start by preheating your oven to 375°F (190°C). Cut the tops off bell peppers and remove the seeds. In a skillet, sauté chopped mushrooms and onions in a small amount of olive oil until tender. Add fresh spinach and cook until wilted. Mix in cooked quinoa or brown rice for added texture and fiber.

Stuff the pepper halves with the spinach and mushroom mixture, place them in a baking dish and bake for 25-30 minutes until the peppers are tender. You can top them with a sprinkle of low-fat cheese if desired. This dish is low in sodium and fat while being rich in vitamins and minerals.

## Chickpea and Sweet Potato Stew

This stew is a comforting and nutritious option. Begin by heating a large pot over medium heat, and adding a tablespoon of olive oil. Sauté onions and garlic until it gets soft. Add diced sweet potatoes, canned chickpeas (drained and rinsed), and vegetable broth. Season with ground cumin, paprika, and a pinch of turmeric. Simmer for 20-25 minutes until the sweet potatoes are tender.

Stir in fresh spinach or kale during the last few minutes of cooking for added nutrients. Adjust the seasoning with salt and pepper to taste. Serve the stew with a side of whole-grain bread or over brown rice for a balanced and heart-healthy meal.

# CHAPTER 9

## Snacking Strategies

### Fresh Fruit and Nut Mix

A fresh fruit and nut mix is a heart-healthy snack that combines the natural sweetness of fruit with the crunchy texture of nuts. To create this mix, select a variety of fresh fruits like apples, pears, and berries. Chop the fruits into bite-sized pieces and mix them with a handful of raw or lightly toasted nuts such as almonds, walnuts, or pistachios. This combination provides essential vitamins, minerals, and healthy fats while keeping sodium and saturated fats low.

For added flavor, sprinkle a dash of cinnamon or a squeeze of lemon juice over the mix. This not only enhances the taste but also adds a hint of extra nutrients. Portion the mix into small containers or resealable bags to make it easy to grab and go, ensuring a quick and healthy snack option that supports cardiovascular health.

## Air-Popped Popcorn with Herbs

Air-popped popcorn is an excellent low-fat snack that can be easily flavored with herbs to boost its taste without adding extra sodium. To make it, use an air popper to pop plain popcorn kernels. Once popped, toss the popcorn with a mixture of dried herbs such as rosemary, thyme, or oregano. You can also add a pinch of garlic powder or paprika for extra flavor.

For a healthier alternative to butter, consider using a light spray of olive oil to help the herbs stick. This method keeps the snack low in fat while providing a satisfying crunch and flavorful experience. Store your seasoned popcorn in an airtight container to maintain freshness and have a heart-friendly snack ready at all times.

# Greek Yogurt with a Drizzle of Honey

Greek yogurt is a versatile ingredient that can be made into a heart-healthy snack by adding a drizzle of honey. Start with plain Greek yogurt, which is low in fat and high in protein. Scoop the yogurt into a bowl and drizzle a small amount of honey on top. Honey adds a natural sweetness without relying on refined sugars, which can be beneficial for heart health.

To increase the nutritional value, consider topping the yogurt with fresh fruit, nuts, or seeds. This not only enhances the flavor but also adds extra fiber and antioxidants, contributing to overall cardiovascular well-being. Enjoy this snack as a quick breakfast or a satisfying afternoon treat.

## Vegetable Sticks with Hummus

Vegetable sticks paired with hummus make for a crunchy and satisfying snack that's also heart-healthy. Cut vegetables such as carrots, celery, cucumbers, and bell peppers into sticks. Prepare or purchase a low-sodium hummus, which provides a creamy and flavorful dip rich in fiber and protein.

Hummus, made from chickpeas, offers essential nutrients while keeping fat and sodium levels in check. This combination of vegetables and hummus is not only convenient and easy to prepare but also supports heart health through its high fiber content and heart-healthy fats. Pack the vegetable sticks and hummus in separate containers for a ready-to-eat snack.

## Roasted Chickpeas

Roasted chickpeas are a crunchy, nutrient-dense snack that can be seasoned to fit heart-healthy dietary guidelines. Rinse and drain a can of chickpeas, then toss them with a small amount of olive oil and your favorite low-sodium spices. Spread the chickpeas on a baking sheet and roast them in the oven at 400°F (200°C) for about 20-30 minutes, shaking the pan occasionally for even cooking.

Once they are crispy and golden, let the chickpeas cool before enjoying them. They offer a satisfying crunch with the added benefit of being high in protein and fiber while being low in saturated fats. Store them in an airtight container to maintain their crispiness and have a convenient snack on hand.

# Chapter 10

# Smoothies

## Berry and Spinach Smoothie

To make a Berry and Spinach Smoothie, blend one cup of fresh spinach with one cup of mixed berries (like strawberries, blueberries, and raspberries). Add half a cup of unsweetened almond milk and a tablespoon of chia seeds for added fiber. Blend until smooth. This combination provides essential vitamins and antioxidants while keeping fat and sodium low, which supports heart health and helps manage blood pressure.

For a sweeter touch, include a small banana or a splash of honey if desired. The berries offer natural sweetness without adding extra sugar, while the spinach adds a nutrient boost. Enjoy this smoothie as a refreshing breakfast or a mid-day snack to keep your heart in check and your taste buds satisfied.

# Tropical Mango and Pineapple Smoothie

Start by blending one cup of fresh or frozen mango chunks with one cup of pineapple chunks. Add half a cup of coconut water for a hydrating base and a squeeze of lime juice for a zesty kick. Blend until smooth and creamy. This smoothie is packed with vitamins A and C, which are beneficial for cardiovascular health and is low in fat and sodium.

If you want to enhance the smoothie's texture, include a tablespoon of flaxseeds or a handful of ice cubes. The mango and pineapple not only provide a tropical flavor but also natural sweetness, making this smoothie a delicious and heart-healthy choice for any time of the day.

## Kale and Kiwi Power Smoothie

To prepare a Kale and Kiwi Power Smoothie, blend one cup of chopped kale with two peeled kiwi fruits. Add half a cup of low-fat yogurt and a tablespoon of honey for sweetness. Blend until well combined. Kale is rich in vitamins K and C, and kiwi provides a good dose of fiber and antioxidants, which are great for heart health.

For a creamier consistency, you can include a small handful of ice or a bit of water if needed. This smoothie provides a nutrient-dense option that supports overall cardiovascular function and helps manage cholesterol levels effectively.

## Apple and Almond Butter Smoothie

For an Apple and Almond Butter Smoothie, blend one medium apple (cored and chopped) with one tablespoon of almond butter and half a cup of unsweetened almond milk. Blend until smooth and creamy. This smoothie combines the fiber from the apple with the healthy fats from the almond butter, which can help reduce cholesterol and support heart health.

If you prefer a thicker texture, add a few ice cubes or a small handful of oats. This smoothie makes for a satisfying and heart-healthy snack or breakfast option, offering a delicious blend of flavors and essential nutrients.

## Banana and Oat Smoothie

To make a Banana and Oat Smoothie, blend one ripe banana with a half-cup of rolled oats and one cup of unsweetened almond milk. Add a sprinkle of cinnamon for extra flavor. Blend until smooth. The banana provides potassium, which helps regulate blood pressure, while the oats offer soluble fiber that aids in lowering cholesterol levels.

For added texture and nutrition, you can incorporate a tablespoon of chia seeds or flaxseeds. This smoothie is a filling and heart-healthy option that helps keep you full while supporting cardiovascular health.

# CHAPTER 11

# Cooking Techniques for Heart Health

## Using Low-Fat Cooking Methods

Low-fat cooking methods are crucial for managing heart disease. Opt for grilling, baking, steaming, and poaching instead of frying. For example, instead of frying chicken, bake it with a light coating of herbs. Steaming vegetables helps retain nutrients while avoiding added fats. Additionally, using a non-stick pan can reduce the need for oil in cooking, thus lowering the fat content in your meals.

Incorporating these methods into your cooking routine can be easy. Start by replacing high-fat ingredients with lower-fat alternatives. For instance, use unsweetened applesauce in place of oil when baking. Embrace techniques like broiling, where fat drips away from the food, helping you to keep your meals healthy and heart-friendly.

## Incorporating Herbs and Spices

Herbs and spices are excellent for enhancing flavor without adding extra sodium or fat. Fresh herbs like basil, cilantro, and parsley can elevate a dish's taste and add nutrients. For example, add a handful of fresh basil to a tomato sauce for a burst of flavor without extra calories. Spices such as cumin, paprika, and garlic powder also contribute robust flavors and can replace salt in recipes.

Experiment with different herb and spice combinations to find what you enjoy most. Creating a seasoning blend with herbs like rosemary and thyme can make grilled vegetables more flavorful. By using these natural flavor enhancers, you can enjoy delicious meals while adhering to a heart-healthy diet.

# Managing Portion Sizes

Managing portion sizes helps control calorie intake and maintain heart health. Use smaller plates and bowls to naturally reduce portion sizes. For instance, serve your main course on a salad plate rather than a dinner plate to visually encourage smaller portions. Additionally, be mindful of serving sizes indicated on nutrition labels to prevent overeating.

Plan meals ahead and use measuring cups to ensure accurate portion sizes. For example, use a ½ cup measuring cup for rice or pasta servings. Portion control also involves listening to your body's hunger cues and avoiding eating out of boredom or stress. Proper portion management helps maintain a balanced diet and supports cardiovascular health.

# Reducing Sodium without Sacrificing Flavor

Reducing sodium can be challenging but is crucial for heart health. Start by cutting back on processed and packaged foods, which often contain high levels of sodium. Opt for fresh ingredients and use salt substitutes or low-sodium versions of your favorite condiments. For instance, try using a salt-free seasoning mix to flavor meats and vegetables.

To further reduce sodium intake, prepare meals from scratch whenever possible. Experiment with homemade sauces and dressings using low-sodium or no-sodium ingredients. For example, make a vinaigrette with lemon juice and herbs instead of a store-bought dressing. These small changes can help keep sodium levels in check while still providing flavorful meals.

# Proper Food Storage and Preparation

Proper food storage and preparation are key to maintaining a heart-healthy diet. Store fresh produce in the refrigerator to preserve its nutrients and extend shelf life. Use airtight containers to keep grains and nuts fresh and avoid spoilage. For example, store whole grains like brown rice in a cool, dry place to prevent rancidity.

When preparing meals, practice safe food handling to prevent contamination. Wash fruits and vegetables thoroughly before use and use separate cutting boards for meats and vegetables to avoid cross-contamination. For example, always use a clean knife and cutting board when prepping chicken to ensure food safety. These practices help ensure that your meals are both healthy and safe.

# CHAPTER 12

# Meal Planning and Prep

## Weekly Meal Planning Tips

Effective weekly meal planning starts with setting aside time each week to outline your meals and snacks. Begin by reviewing your week's schedule to identify busy days when quick meals are essential. Choose recipes that align with heart-healthy principles, such as those low in fat and sodium. Create a meal plan that includes breakfast, lunch, dinner, and snacks to ensure balanced nutrition throughout the week.

Once your plan is in place, make a shopping list based on the ingredients needed for each meal. This helps avoid last-minute trips to the store and reduces impulse buys. Utilize digital tools or apps to organize your plan and shopping list efficiently. For variety and sustainability, incorporate seasonal fruits and vegetables into your weekly plan.

## Creating a Balanced Grocery List

A balanced grocery list starts with selecting whole, unprocessed foods. Focus on purchasing fresh vegetables, fruits, lean proteins (like chicken or fish), whole grains, and low-fat dairy products. Avoid processed foods high in sodium and unhealthy fats by reading labels and opting for items with minimal added sugars and sodium.

To ensure a heart-healthy diet, include staples such as beans, lentils, and nuts which are high in fiber and beneficial fats. Incorporate herbs and spices for flavoring instead of salt. Organizing your list by food categories—produce, proteins, grains—can streamline your shopping and make it easier to stick to your nutritional goals.

# Preparing Meals in Advance

Meal prep involves cooking and portioning meals ahead of time to save effort during the week. Start by choosing recipes that can be made in batches, such as soups, stews, or casseroles. Prepare these meals in large quantities and store them in individual portions for easy access.

Use clear, airtight containers to keep prepped meals fresh. Label each container with the date to ensure you consume them within a safe period. Freezing some of these meals can also extend their shelf life and provide convenient options for busy days.

# Portion Control and Storage

Portion control is key to managing calorie intake and maintaining a heart-healthy diet. Use measuring cups or a food scale to portion out meals according to dietary guidelines. Aim to fill half your plate with vegetables, a quarter with lean protein, and a quarter with whole grains.

Proper storage is crucial to maintain the quality and safety of your meals. Refrigerate perishable items promptly and keep your fridge at 40°F (4°C) or below. For longer storage, use freezer-safe bags or containers and label them with dates to prevent freezer burn and ensure you use them within a recommended time frame.

## Quick and Easy Meal Ideas

Quick and easy heart-healthy meals include dishes that require minimal preparation and cooking time. For breakfast, try Greek yogurt with fresh berries and a sprinkle of flaxseed. For lunch, prepare a salad with mixed greens, cherry tomatoes, grilled chicken, and a light vinaigrette.

For dinner, consider a one-pan dish such as baked salmon with steamed broccoli and quinoa. Utilize slow cookers or pressure cookers for convenient, hands-off cooking. Keep frozen vegetables and pre-cooked beans on hand to quickly assemble nutritious meals.

# CHAPTER 13

# Understanding Labels and Ingredients

## Reading Nutrition Labels Effectively

Nutrition labels are crucial for managing heart health. Start by checking the "Serving Size" to ensure you're not consuming more than you intend. Pay attention to the "Total Fat" and "Sodium" sections—aim for products with lower amounts of these components. For fat, look for less than 5 grams per serving, and for sodium, ideally less than 140 milligrams per serving. Remember, even seemingly small amounts can add up over the course of the day.

Also, consider the "Percent Daily Value" which shows how a serving of the product contributes to your daily nutritional needs. Focus on foods with lower percentages of saturated fat and sodium. For example, choose cereals with less than 10% of the daily value for sodium and saturated fat. This helps you select items that align with heart-healthy goals without sacrificing flavor or variety.

## Identifying Hidden Sources of Sodium and Fat

Hidden sodium and fat can be found in many processed and packaged foods. For instance, sauces, dressings, and even bread can contain significant amounts of sodium and fat. Always check the labels of these items, even if they appear healthy, to avoid unknowingly increasing your intake.

Another common source is fast food and restaurant meals. Opt for grilled or baked options instead of fried, and ask for dressings or sauces on the side. This way, you can control the amount added and avoid excessive sodium and fat intake that often accompanies restaurant servings.

# Understanding Ingredient Lists

The ingredient list on food packaging provides insight into the content of the product. Ingredients are listed in descending order by weight, so the first few ingredients are the most prevalent. For heart health, avoid products where "sodium" or "saturated fat" are listed among the first few ingredients.

Watch out for ingredients like "hydrogenated oils" or "partially hydrogenated oils," which indicate the presence of trans fats. These unhealthy fats can raise cholesterol levels and increase heart disease risk. Opt for products where these terms are absent, and instead, look for items with healthier fats such as olive oil or avocado oil listed.

# Choosing Heart-Healthy Alternatives

Opting for heart-healthy alternatives involves selecting foods low in saturated fat, cholesterol, and sodium. For example, choose lean meats like chicken breast instead of fatty cuts of beef or pork. Replace butter with olive oil or avocado for cooking, as these fats are better for heart health.

Whole grains are another excellent choice. Swap white rice or bread with whole grain options like brown rice or whole wheat bread. These alternatives provide more fiber and nutrients that help in reducing cholesterol levels and improving overall cardiovascular health.

## Common Misleading Terms to Avoid

Certain terms on food packaging can be misleading. For instance, "low-fat" does not necessarily mean low in sodium or cholesterol. Similarly, "natural" does not equate to heart-healthy. Always cross-reference these claims with the actual nutrition label to ensure the product meets your dietary needs.

Be cautious with "sugar-free" or "fat-free" products as they may contain high amounts of sodium or artificial additives. Instead, focus on the overall nutritional profile and select products with balanced and wholesome ingredients that align with heart-healthy eating patterns.

# CHAPTER 14

# <u>Adjusting Recipes for</u>
# <u>Heart Health</u>

## Modifying Traditional Recipes

When adapting traditional recipes for heart health, focus on reducing fat and sodium without sacrificing flavor. For instance, use skinless chicken instead of fatty cuts and swap heavy cream with low-fat yogurt or milk. To enhance the texture, try baking or grilling rather than frying, and adjust cooking times as needed. By making these simple changes, you can maintain the essence of your favorite dishes while aligning them with heart-healthy guidelines.

Another approach is to incorporate more vegetables and legumes into your recipes. These ingredients are naturally low in fat and high in fiber, which can help lower cholesterol and blood pressure. For example, replace half of the ground beef in a meatloaf with lentils or mushrooms. This not only reduces fat content but also adds additional nutrients and flavors.

## Substituting Ingredients for Lower Fat and Sodium

Substitute high-fat ingredients with heart-healthy alternatives to make your meals more nutritious. For example, replace butter with olive oil or avocado in recipes. Olive oil contains monounsaturated fats, which are better for heart health. Similarly, use low-sodium or no-salt-added versions of canned goods and broths to cut down on sodium intake.

To reduce sodium, season your dishes with herbs and spices rather than salt. Fresh or dried herbs like basil, oregano, and thyme can add robust flavors to your meals without the extra sodium. For example, instead of adding salt to a pasta dish, try seasoning it with garlic, black pepper, and fresh basil for a delicious and heart-healthy alternative.

# Reducing Sugar and Refined Carbs

Cutting down on sugar and refined carbs is crucial for maintaining cardiovascular health. Opt for whole grains such as brown rice, quinoa, and whole-wheat pasta instead of refined grains. These whole grains provide more fiber and nutrients, which help manage blood sugar levels and improve heart health.

In baking, replace white sugar with natural sweeteners like applesauce or mashed bananas. These alternatives add moisture and sweetness with fewer calories and less sugar. For instance, if a recipe calls for one cup of sugar, you might use half a cup of applesauce along with a quarter cup of honey to maintain the texture and flavor while reducing sugar content.

# Flavor Enhancements without Extra Salt

Enhance the flavor of your meals without relying on extra salt by using various flavoring techniques. Incorporate a variety of herbs, spices, and citrus juices to create depth and complexity in your dishes. For example, adding lemon zest or a splash of balsamic vinegar can brighten up a dish and replace the need for salt.

Experiment with spice blends and marinades that emphasize natural flavors. Create a spice mix with ingredients like paprika, cumin, and coriander to season meats and vegetables. These blends can provide a flavorful punch without increasing sodium content, making your meals both enjoyable and heart-healthy.

## Tips for Baking Healthier Treats

When baking treats, opt for whole-grain flour like whole wheat or oat flour to increase fiber content.

Additionally, reduce the amount of sugar in recipes and use healthier substitutes such as honey or maple syrup. For example, if a cookie recipe calls for one cup of sugar, you can cut it down to half a cup and add a tablespoon of honey to maintain sweetness.

Incorporate healthy fats such as nuts, seeds, or avocado into your baked goods. These ingredients provide essential fatty acids that are beneficial for heart health. For instance, adding chopped walnuts to muffins not only enhances texture but also contributes to a healthier fat profile. Experiment with these substitutions to enjoy delicious treats that support cardiovascular well-being.

# CHAPTER 15

## Special Dietary Needs

### Managing Diabetes and Heart Disease Together

Balancing diabetes and heart disease requires a careful selection of foods that manage blood sugar while promoting cardiovascular health. Focus on meals rich in fiber, such as whole grains, legumes, and vegetables, which help stabilize blood sugar and reduce cholesterol levels. For instance, a salad with quinoa, black beans, and a variety of colorful veggies provides essential nutrients and keeps blood sugar levels steady.

Incorporate lean proteins like chicken breast or fish and healthy fats from sources such as avocados and nuts. Limit added sugars and refined carbs to control blood glucose levels, and opt for heart-healthy cooking methods such as grilling or baking instead of frying. For a practical meal, try a grilled chicken breast with a side of roasted Brussels sprouts and a quinoa salad for a balanced, low-fat, and diabetes-friendly option.

## Gluten-Free Options

For those needing gluten-free meals, focus on naturally gluten-free grains like rice, quinoa, and buckwheat. These grains are excellent for heart health as they are low in fat and high in fiber. For example, a quinoa-stuffed bell pepper or a bowl of brown rice with mixed vegetables offers a nutritious, gluten-free option that supports cardiovascular well-being.

Use gluten-free flour such as almond or coconut flour for baking and cooking. These alternatives provide essential nutrients while keeping your diet heart-healthy. A gluten-free banana bread made with almond flour, or gluten-free oats in a breakfast porridge, ensures you enjoy tasty, safe meals without compromising your heart health.

## Low-Carb Heart-Healthy Choices

Low-carb diets can support heart health by reducing saturated fat and cholesterol levels. Opt for non-starchy vegetables like leafy greens, peppers, and cucumbers, which are low in carbs and high in essential vitamins. A simple dish could be a spinach and mushroom omelet, which is both low in carbs and high in heart-healthy nutrients.

Replace high-carb foods with protein-rich options such as eggs, tofu, or lean meats. For example, a grilled salmon fillet with a side of steamed broccoli offers a heart-healthy, low-carb meal that helps manage weight and promotes cardiovascular health. Emphasize lean proteins and low-carb vegetables to maintain heart health while adhering to a low-carb lifestyle.

# Vegetarian and Vegan Adjustments

Vegetarian and vegan diets can be heart-healthy by focusing on plant-based proteins and fiber-rich foods. Include legumes like lentils, chickpeas, and black beans in your meals. A hearty lentil stew with carrots and celery provides essential nutrients and supports heart health while being entirely plant-based.

Ensure you're getting enough omega-3 fatty acids from sources like chia seeds, flaxseeds, and walnuts, which are crucial for heart health. A salad with mixed greens, walnuts, and a flaxseed dressing makes a nutritious, vegan-friendly meal that supports cardiovascular well-being. Embrace a variety of vegetables, whole grains, and plant-based proteins to create balanced, heart-healthy meals.

# Allergy-Friendly Recipe Adaptations

Adapting recipes to be allergy-friendly involves substituting common allergens with safe alternatives. For dairy allergies, use almond or coconut milk instead of cow's milk in recipes. For example, a smoothie made with almond milk, spinach, and berries is both allergy-friendly and heart-healthy.

When dealing with nut allergies, use seeds like pumpkin or sunflower seeds for added crunch and nutrients. A sunflower seed granola or a chia seed pudding can replace recipes that typically use nuts, providing similar texture and nutritional benefits while being safe for those with nut allergies. Tailor your recipes to include safe, nutritious alternatives that cater to specific dietary needs while promoting heart health.

# CHAPTER 16

# Integrating Exercise with Diet

## Benefits of Regular Physical Activity

Regular physical activity is essential for maintaining cardiovascular health. Engaging in activities like brisk walking, cycling, or swimming helps improve heart function by enhancing blood circulation and reducing blood pressure. Consistent exercise also aids in lowering LDL cholesterol levels while boosting HDL cholesterol, which is beneficial for heart health. Additionally, physical activity helps manage weight, reducing the risk of obesity-related heart disease.

Beyond cardiovascular benefits, regular exercise improves overall well-being. It supports mental health by reducing stress and anxiety, promoting better sleep, and increasing energy levels. Exercise also strengthens muscles and bones, which can help prevent injuries and improve mobility, contributing to a healthier lifestyle.

## Combining Diet and Exercise for Optimal Health

To achieve optimal cardiovascular health, combining a heart-healthy diet with regular exercise is crucial. A diet low in saturated fats and sodium, rich in fruits, vegetables, whole grains, and lean proteins, complements the benefits of physical activity. Eating nutrient-dense foods helps manage weight, control blood pressure, and reduce cholesterol levels, all of which support heart health.

Incorporating exercise routines that align with dietary goals further enhances cardiovascular benefits. For instance, pairing a low-sodium diet with activities like jogging or strength training helps to maintain a healthy weight and improve overall heart function. The synergy between diet and exercise maximizes health benefits, making it easier to achieve and maintain a healthy lifestyle.

## Simple Exercises for Beginners

For beginners, starting with simple exercises can ease the transition into a regular workout routine. Walking at a brisk pace is an excellent starting point; it's low-impact and easily adaptable to different fitness levels. Other beginner-friendly exercises include gentle stretching, chair exercises, and basic bodyweight exercises like squats and wall push-ups.

Gradually increasing intensity and duration helps build endurance and strength. Aim for short, manageable sessions and gradually progress as fitness improves. Consistency is key, so find enjoyable activities and incorporate them into your routine to maintain motivation and ensure long-term success.

# Incorporating Activity into Daily Routines

Integrating physical activity into daily routines can significantly enhance overall fitness without requiring extra time. Simple strategies include taking the stairs instead of the elevator, walking or biking to work, or performing short exercise breaks during the day. Activities like gardening, cleaning, or playing with pets also contribute to daily physical activity.

To make it easier, identify opportunities for movement throughout the day. For example, standing or using a stability ball at your desk can help reduce sedentary time. Small, consistent changes lead to improved cardiovascular health and increased overall activity levels.

Setting Realistic Fitness Goals

Setting realistic fitness goals is essential for maintaining motivation and achieving long-term success. Begin by defining specific, achievable objectives, such as walking for 20 minutes a day or gradually increasing the weight used in strength training. Break larger goals into smaller, manageable steps to track progress and celebrate achievements along the way.

Ensure that goals are tailored to your fitness level and health needs. Setting incremental targets and adjusting them as needed helps maintain focus and adaptability. Remember, consistency and gradual progress are key to achieving and sustaining fitness goals effectively.

# CHAPTER 17

# Maintaining Long-Term Heart Health

## Setting and Tracking Dietary Goals

Begin by identifying specific dietary goals that align with heart health, such as reducing sodium intake or increasing fiber consumption. Create a detailed plan with clear, actionable steps, like choosing low-fat, low-sodium recipes and substituting high-cholesterol ingredients with healthier alternatives. Use a food diary or a mobile app to log daily meals, making note of nutrient intake and comparing it to your goals.

To effectively track your progress, regularly review your food diary and adjust your diet as needed. Set short-term milestones, such as achieving a certain number of low-sodium meals per week, and monitor changes in your blood pressure and cholesterol levels. Regularly assessing these metrics will help you stay on track and make necessary adjustments to reach your dietary goals.

## Overcoming Common Challenges

One common challenge is dealing with cravings for high-fat or high-sodium foods. Combat this by finding satisfying, heart-healthy substitutes, like using herbs and spices to enhance flavor without adding extra sodium. Planning and preparing meals in advance can also help avoid the temptation of unhealthy choices when hunger strikes.

Another challenge is managing time constraints. To overcome this, focus on quick and easy recipes that require minimal preparation and cooking time. Batch cooking and using meal prep techniques can streamline the process, ensuring that healthy, heart-friendly options are always available when you need them.

## Staying Motivated and Consistent

Maintaining motivation involves setting realistic goals and celebrating small victories along the way. Keep a journal of your progress and acknowledge improvements, whether it's a reduction in cholesterol levels or successfully trying a new heart-healthy recipe. Reward yourself with non-food-related treats, such as a relaxing activity or a new kitchen gadget.

Consistency is key to long-term success. Create a routine by scheduling regular meal times and planning weekly menus. Building healthy habits, like meal prepping on weekends or involving family members in cooking, can make it easier to stick to your dietary plan and maintain a heart-healthy lifestyle.

# Finding Support and Resources

Leverage support from healthcare professionals, such as dietitians or nutritionists, who can offer personalized advice and guidance. Joining a support group for individuals with similar dietary goals can provide motivation and share practical tips. Online forums and social media groups can also be valuable resources for recipes and encouragement.

Utilize reputable resources, such as heart health cookbooks and websites, to access a variety of low-fat, low-sodium recipes. Educational materials from organizations like the American Heart Association can offer further insights into managing heart disease through diet. Having these resources at your disposal can make it easier to stay informed and committed to your health goals.

# Celebrating Milestones and Successes

Recognize and celebrate milestones, such as achieving a target reduction in cholesterol levels or successfully maintaining a heart-healthy diet for a month. Hosting a small gathering with friends or family to showcase your cooking achievements can be a fun way to celebrate. Share your progress and successes with others to inspire and motivate them.

Set new goals and challenges to continue progressing in your heart health journey. Each success, whether big or small, should be acknowledged and used as motivation to keep improving. Regularly reflecting on your achievements can boost confidence and reinforce your commitment to a heart-healthy lifestyle.

# CHAPTER 18:

# Common Concerns and Detailed FAQs

## How to Deal with Cravings for Unhealthy Foods

When dealing with cravings for unhealthy foods, it's essential to identify healthier alternatives that satisfy your taste buds. For example, if you're craving salty snacks, try air-popped popcorn seasoned with a sprinkle of herbs instead of chips. Keeping nutritious snacks like fruits, nuts, or yogurt readily available can also help manage cravings. Additionally, staying hydrated and incorporating more fiber-rich foods into your diet can reduce the frequency and intensity of these cravings.

Practicing mindful eating can also aid in overcoming cravings. Slow down and savor each bite, which can help you feel more satisfied with smaller portions of healthier options. If a craving persists, consider distraction techniques such as engaging in a hobby, exercising, or simply taking a walk. By using these strategies, you can better manage cravings without resorting to unhealthy choices.

## Managing Eating Out and Social Situations

Navigating restaurant menus and social events while sticking to a heart-healthy diet can be challenging. Start by researching restaurant menus online before dining out to identify healthier options. Opt for dishes that are grilled, baked, or steamed, and ask for dressings or sauces on the side to control sodium and fat intake. Choosing meals that include plenty of vegetables, lean proteins, and whole grains can align with your dietary goals.

In social settings, don't hesitate to communicate your dietary needs to hosts or servers. Many restaurants and hosts are accommodating if you inform them of your heart-healthy requirements. Bring a heart-healthy dish to potlucks or gatherings to ensure there's something suitable for you to enjoy. By planning ahead and making thoughtful choices, you can maintain your dietary goals without feeling deprived in social situations.

## Adjusting Recipes for Family Preferences

Adjusting recipes to meet family preferences while adhering to heart-healthy guidelines involves simple modifications. For instance, replace high-fat meats with lean proteins like chicken or turkey, and use herbs and spices for flavor instead of salt. If a family favorite calls for cream, substitute it with low-fat yogurt or plant-based milk to cut down on saturated fat.

Incorporate more vegetables and whole grains into your recipes, which can enhance nutrition without compromising taste. When baking, use applesauce or mashed bananas as substitutes for butter or oil.

By making these changes, you can create meals that are both heart-healthy and enjoyable for the whole family.

## Handling Dietary Changes with a Busy Lifestyle

Managing a heart-healthy diet with a busy schedule requires strategic planning and preparation. Batch cooking on weekends or your days off can save time during the week. Prepare and freeze meals like soups, stews, or casseroles in portioned containers to have ready-to-eat options that align with your dietary goals.

Utilize quick and nutritious recipes that require minimal preparation, such as salads with pre-cooked proteins or overnight oats. Having a selection of healthy, easy-to-grab snacks like cut-up vegetables, fruit, or whole-grain crackers can also help you stay on track even on the busiest days.

## Addressing Misconceptions about Heart-Healthy Eating

One common misconception about heart-healthy eating is that it's bland and unappetizing. In reality, heart-healthy meals can be flavorful and satisfying by using a variety of herbs, spices, and fresh ingredients. For instance, lemon juice and garlic can enhance the taste of grilled fish, making it both heart-healthy and delicious.

Another misconception is that heart-healthy eating is expensive. With careful planning, you can eat healthily on a budget by purchasing seasonal vegetables, buying in bulk, and choosing less expensive protein sources like beans and lentils. Educating yourself about cost-effective, nutritious options helps dispel these myths and supports a heart-healthy lifestyle.

# CHAPTER 19

# <u>Resources and Further Reading</u>

## Online Resources and Tools

Numerous online resources are available to assist with managing heart disease through diet. Some Websites provide access to free tools, including meal planners and heart-healthy recipe databases. Interactive tools on these sites allow users to input their dietary preferences and health goals to generate personalized meal plans that align with heart disease management principles.

Most Apps can also be useful. These applications allow users to track their food intake, monitor sodium and fat consumption, and receive personalized feedback. By logging meals and snacks, users can easily stay on top of their dietary goals and make adjustments as needed, making heart-healthy eating more manageable.

## Support Groups and Forums

Support groups and forums provide a valuable community for individuals managing heart disease. Some Online forums are dedicated to sharing heart health experiences, recipes, and tips. Engaging in these communities can provide emotional support, practical advice, and motivation from others facing similar challenges.

Local support groups also play a crucial role. Many hospitals and community centers host meetings where individuals can discuss dietary strategies, share successes, and seek advice from peers. These groups often feature guest speakers, such as dietitians or cardiologists, who provide expert insights and answer questions about heart-healthy living.

# Cooking Classes and Workshops

Cooking classes and workshops focused on heart-healthy cooking can greatly simplify the process of adopting a new diet. Local community centers, hospitals, and culinary schools often offer classes that teach how to prepare low-fat, low-sodium meals. These classes provide hands-on experience with ingredient selection, meal preparation techniques, and cooking methods that align with heart health guidelines.

Online workshops are also available, offering virtual cooking demonstrations and interactive sessions. Some Websites feature courses on heart-healthy cooking, allowing participants to learn at their own pace. These workshops often include detailed recipes and cooking tips, making it easier for beginners to practice and master heart-healthy cooking techniques at home.

# 3 weeks Meal Plan Recipes, Ingredients and their Preparation procedures

## DAY 1: Grilled Chicken Salad with Lemon Vinaigrette

**Ingredients:**

5. 2 boneless, skinless chicken breasts
6. 4 cups mixed greens (e.g., spinach, arugula, romaine)
7. 1 cup cherry tomatoes, halved
8. 1 cucumber, sliced
9. 1/2 red onion, thinly sliced
10. 1/4 cup feta cheese, crumbled (optional)
11. 2 tablespoons olive oil
12. 2 tablespoons lemon juice
13. 1 teaspoon Dijon mustard
14. Salt and pepper to taste

**Preparation:**

1. Preheat the grill to medium-high heat. Season chicken breasts with salt and pepper.
2. Grill chicken for 6-7 minutes per side, or until fully cooked. Let rest before slicing.
3. In a large bowl, combine mixed greens, cherry tomatoes, cucumber, and red onion.
4. Slice the grilled chicken and place it on top of the salad.
5. For the vinaigrette, whisk together olive oil, lemon juice, Dijon mustard, salt, and pepper.
6. Drizzle vinaigrette over the salad and top with feta cheese if using.

# DAY 2: Baked Salmon with Asparagus and Quinoa

**Ingredients:**

1. 2 salmon fillets
2. 1 bunch asparagus, trimmed
3. 1 tablespoon olive oil

4. 1 lemon, sliced

5. 1 teaspoon dried dill

6. 1 cup quinoa

7. 2 cups water or low-sodium vegetable broth

8. Salt and pepper to taste

## Preparation:

1. Preheat oven to 375°F (190°C). Place salmon fillets on a baking sheet lined with parchment paper.

2. Drizzle salmon with olive oil, and season with dill, salt, and pepper. Place lemon slices on top.

3. Arrange asparagus around the salmon on the baking sheet. Drizzle with a little olive oil.

4. Bake for 15-20 minutes or until salmon flakes easily with a fork.

5. While salmon and asparagus bake, rinse quinoa under cold water.

6. In a saucepan, bring water or broth to a boil. Add quinoa, reduce heat, cover, and simmer for 15 minutes. Fluff with a fork.

# DAY 3: Turkey and Vegetable Stir-Fry

**Ingredients:**

1. 1 pound ground turkey
2. 2 cups broccoli florets
3. 1 bell pepper, sliced
4. 1 carrot, sliced
5. 2 tablespoons low-sodium soy sauce
6. 1 tablespoon olive oil
7. 1 teaspoon minced garlic
8. 1 teaspoon minced ginger
9. 1 tablespoon cornstarch mixed with 2 tablespoons water (optional for thickening)

**Preparation:**

1. Heat olive oil in a large skillet over medium heat. Add garlic and ginger, and cook for 1 minute.
2. Add ground turkey and cook until browned, breaking it up with a spoon.
3. Add broccoli, bell pepper, and carrot. Stir-fry for 5-7 minutes until vegetables are tender.
4. Stir in soy sauce. If using cornstarch, add the mixture to thicken the sauce.
5. Cook for an additional 2 minutes, then serve.

# DAY 4: Lentil and Spinach Soup

**Ingredients:**

1. 1 cup dried lentils, rinsed
2. 4 cups low-sodium vegetable broth
3. 1 cup fresh spinach, chopped
4. 1 onion, diced
5. 2 carrots, diced
6. 2 celery stalks, diced

7. 2 cloves garlic, minced

8. 1 tablespoon olive oil

9. 1 teaspoon dried thyme

10.　　Salt and pepper to taste

## Preparation:

1. In a large pot, heat olive oil over medium heat. Add onion, carrots, and celery, and cook until softened.

2. Add garlic and thyme, and cook for 1 minute.

3. Add lentils and vegetable broth. Bring to a boil, then reduce heat and simmer for 25 minutes.

4. Stir in spinach and cook for an additional 5 minutes.

5. Season with salt and pepper to taste before serving.

# DAY 5: Quinoa-Stuffed Bell Peppers

**Ingredients:**

1. 4 bell peppers (any color)
2. 1 cup cooked quinoa
3. 1 cup black beans, rinsed
4. 1 cup corn kernels
5. 1 cup diced tomatoes
6. 1 teaspoon cumin
7. 1 teaspoon paprika
8. 1/2 cup shredded low-fat cheese (optional)
9. Salt and pepper to taste

**Preparation:**

1. Preheat oven to 375°F (190°C). Cut the tops off the bell peppers and remove the seeds.
2. In a bowl, combine quinoa, black beans, corn, diced tomatoes, cumin, paprika, salt, and pepper.
3. Stuff each pepper with the quinoa mixture.

4. Place stuffed peppers in a baking dish. If using cheese, sprinkle on top.
5. Bake for 30 minutes or until peppers are tender.

# DAY 6: Spaghetti Squash with Tomato Basil Sauce

## Ingredients:

1. 1 large spaghetti squash
2. 2 cups canned crushed tomatoes
3. 1 onion, diced
4. 2 cloves garlic, minced
5. 1 tablespoon olive oil
6. 1 teaspoon dried basil
7. 1 teaspoon dried oregano
8. Salt and pepper to taste

## Preparation:

1. Preheat oven to 400°F (200°C). Cut spaghetti squash in half and remove seeds. Place cut-side down on a baking sheet.

2. Bake for 40-45 minutes, or until tender. Use a fork to scrape out spaghetti-like strands.

3. In a skillet, heat olive oil over medium heat. Add onion and garlic, and cook until softened.

4. Stir in crushed tomatoes, basil, oregano, salt, and pepper. Simmer for 10 minutes.

5. Toss spaghetti squash with tomato sauce before serving.

# DAY 7: Chickpea and Avocado Salad

## Ingredients:

1. 1 can chickpeas, drained and rinsed
2. 1 avocado, diced
3. 1 cup cherry tomatoes, halved
4. 1/2 red onion, diced

5. 2 tablespoons olive oil

6. 1 tablespoon lemon juice

7. 1 teaspoon ground cumin

8. Salt and pepper to taste

## Preparation:

1. In a large bowl, combine chickpeas, avocado, cherry tomatoes, and red onion.

2. In a small bowl, whisk together olive oil, lemon juice, cumin, salt, and pepper.

3. Pour dressing over the salad and toss gently.

# DAY 8: Stuffed Sweet Potatoes

## Ingredients:

1. 4 medium sweet potatoes

2. 1 cup cooked black beans

3. 1 cup corn kernels

4. 1/2 cup salsa

5. 1/2 teaspoon chili powder

6. 1/2 teaspoon cumin

7. Salt and pepper to taste

**Preparation:**

1. Preheat oven to 400°F (200°C). Pierce sweet potatoes with a fork and place on a baking sheet.
2. Bake for 45-60 minutes, or until tender.
3. In a bowl, mix black beans, corn, salsa, chili powder, cumin, salt, and pepper.
4. Once sweet potatoes are cooked, cut them open and fluff the insides with a fork. Stuff with the black bean mixture.

# DAY 9: Chicken and Vegetable Skewers

**Ingredients:**

1. 2 boneless, skinless chicken breasts, cut into cubes
2. 1 zucchini, sliced
3. 1 red bell pepper, cut into chunks
4. 1 onion, cut into chunks
5. 2 tablespoons olive oil

6. 1 tablespoon lemon juice

7. 1 teaspoon dried oregano

8. Salt and pepper to taste

## Preparation:

1. Preheat the grill to medium-high heat.

2. In a bowl, mix olive oil, lemon juice, oregano, salt, and pepper. Toss chicken cubes in the marinade.

3. Thread chicken, zucchini, bell pepper, and onion onto skewers.

4. Grill skewers for 10-15 minutes, turning occasionally, until chicken is cooked through.

# DAY 10: Turkey and Spinach Stuffed Mushrooms

## Ingredients:

1. 12 large mushrooms, stems removed

2. 1/2 pound ground turkey

3. 1 cup fresh spinach, chopped

4. 1/4 cup onion, finely chopped

5. 1 garlic clove, minced
6. 1 tablespoon olive oil
7. 1/4 cup breadcrumbs (optional)
8. Salt and pepper to taste

## Preparation:

1. Preheat oven to 375°F (190°C).
2. Heat olive oil in a skillet over medium heat. Add onion and garlic, and cook until softened.
3. Add ground turkey and cook until browned. Stir in spinach and cook until wilted.
4. Season with salt and pepper. If using breadcrumbs, mix in for texture.
5. Stuff mushroom caps with the turkey mixture and place on a baking sheet.
6. Bake for 15-20 minutes, until mushrooms are tender.

## DAY 11: Cauliflower Fried Rice

### Ingredients:

1. 1 head cauliflower, grated or processed into rice-sized pieces
2. 1 cup frozen peas and carrots
3. 2 eggs, beaten
4. 2 tablespoons low-sodium soy sauce
5. 1 tablespoon olive oil
6. 2 cloves garlic, minced
7. 1/2 onion, diced

**Preparation:**

1. Heat olive oil in a large skillet or wok over medium heat. Add garlic and onion, and cook until softened.
2. Add peas and carrots and cook for 3-4 minutes.
3. Push vegetables to one side of the skillet. Pour beaten eggs into the empty side and scramble until cooked.
4. Add the cauliflower "rice" and soy sauce. Stir to combine and cook for 5-7 minutes.

# DAY 12: Greek Yogurt Chicken Salad

## Ingredients:

1. 2 cooked chicken breasts, shredded
2. 1/2 cup plain Greek yogurt
3. 1 tablespoon lemon juice
4. 1 tablespoon Dijon mustard
5. 1 celery stalk, diced
6. 1/4 cup red grapes, halved
7. 1/4 cup walnuts, chopped (optional)
8. Salt and pepper to taste

## Preparation:

1. In a bowl, combine Greek yogurt, lemon juice, Dijon mustard, salt, and pepper.
2. Add shredded chicken, celery, grapes, and walnuts. Mix until well combined.
3. Chill before serving.

# DAY 13: Zucchini Noodles with Pesto

## Ingredients:

1. 4 medium zucchinis, Spiralized into noodles
2. 1/4 cup fresh basil leaves
3. 1/4 cup pine nuts
4. 2 cloves garlic
5. 1/4 cup grated Parmesan cheese (optional)
6. 1/4 cup olive oil
7. Salt and pepper to taste

## Preparation:

1. In a food processor, combine basil, pine nuts, garlic, Parmesan (if using), and olive oil. Blend until smooth.
2. Toss zucchini noodles with pesto sauce.
3. Serve immediately or chilled.

# DAY 14: Black Bean and Corn Salad

## Ingredients:

1. 1 can black beans, drained and rinsed
2. 1 cup corn kernels
3. 1 red bell pepper, diced
4. 1/2 red onion, diced
5. 1/4 cup cilantro, chopped
6. 2 tablespoons lime juice
7. 1 tablespoon olive oil
8. Salt and pepper to taste

## Preparation:

1. In a large bowl, combine black beans, corn, bell pepper, red onion, and cilantro.
2. In a small bowl, whisk together lime juice, olive oil, salt, and pepper.
3. Pour dressing over the salad and toss to combine.

# DAY 15: Baked Cod with Lemon and Dill

## Ingredients:

1. 2 cod fillets
2. 1 lemon, thinly sliced
3. 1 tablespoon olive oil
4. 1 teaspoon dried dill
5. Salt and pepper to taste

## Preparation:

1. Preheat oven to 375°F (190°C). Place cod fillets on a baking sheet lined with parchment paper.
2. Drizzle with olive oil and season with dill, salt, and pepper. Place lemon slices on top of the cod.
3. Bake for 15-20 minutes or until the fish flakes easily with a fork.

# DAY 16: Spinach and Mushroom Stuffed Chicken Breast

## Ingredients:

1. 2 boneless, skinless chicken breasts
2. 1 cup fresh spinach, chopped
3. 1/2 cup mushrooms, diced
4. 1 garlic clove, minced
5. 1 tablespoon olive oil
6. 1/4 cup low-fat cream cheese (optional)
7. Salt and pepper to taste

## Preparation:

1. Preheat oven to 375°F (190°C).
2. In a skillet, heat olive oil over medium heat. Add garlic and mushrooms, and cook until mushrooms are tender.
3. Stir in spinach and cook until wilted. Remove from heat and mix in cream cheese if using.
4. Cut a pocket into each chicken breast and stuff with the spinach mixture.

5. Season the outside of the chicken with salt and pepper. Place on a baking sheet and bake for 25-30 minutes, until chicken is cooked through.

# DAY 17: Sweet Potato and Black Bean Chili

**Ingredients:**

1. 2 large sweet potatoes, peeled and diced
2. 1 can black beans, drained and rinsed
3. 1 can diced tomatoes
4. 1 cup corn kernels
5. 1 onion, diced
6. 2 cloves garlic, minced
7. 2 tablespoons chili powder
8. 1 teaspoon cumin
9. 1 tablespoon olive oil
10. Salt and pepper to taste

## Preparation:

1. Heat olive oil in a large pot over medium heat. Add onion and garlic, and cook until softened.

2. Stir in chili powder and cumin, and cook for 1 minute.

3. Add sweet potatoes, black beans, diced tomatoes, and corn. Bring to a boil.

4. Reduce heat, cover, and simmer for 25-30 minutes, until sweet potatoes are tender.

5. Season with salt and pepper to taste before serving.

# DAY 18: Mediterranean Chickpea Bowl

## Ingredients:

1. 1 can chickpeas, drained and rinsed
2. 1 cup cherry tomatoes, halved
3. 1 cucumber, diced
4. 1/4 cup Kalamata olives, sliced
5. 1/4 cup red onion, diced

6. 2 tablespoons olive oil

7. 2 tablespoons red wine vinegar

8. 1 teaspoon dried oregano

9. Salt and pepper to taste

## Preparation:

1. In a large bowl, combine chickpeas, cherry tomatoes, cucumber, olives, and red onion.

2. In a small bowl, whisk together olive oil, red wine vinegar, oregano, salt, and pepper.

3. Pour dressing over the chickpea mixture and toss to combine.

# DAY 19: Cauliflower and Chickpea Curry

## Ingredients:

1. 1 head cauliflower, cut into florets

2. 1 can chickpeas, drained and rinsed

3. 1 can coconut milk (light)

4. 1 onion, diced

5. 2 cloves garlic, minced

6. 1 tablespoon curry powder

7. 1 teaspoon turmeric

8. 1 tablespoon olive oil

9. Salt and pepper to taste

## Preparation:

1. Heat olive oil in a large skillet over medium heat. Add onion and garlic, and cook until softened.

2. Stir in curry powder and turmeric, and cook for 1 minute.

3. Add cauliflower florets, chickpeas, and coconut milk. Bring to a simmer.

4. Cover and cook for 15-20 minutes, until cauliflower is tender.

5. Season with salt and pepper to taste before serving.

# DAY 20: Turkey and Spinach Meatballs

## Ingredients:

1. 1 pound ground turkey
2. 1 cup fresh spinach, finely chopped
3. 1/4 cup breadcrumbs (optional)
4. 1 egg, beaten
5. 1 teaspoon dried oregano
6. 1 teaspoon garlic powder
7. 1/2 teaspoon onion powder
8. Salt and pepper to taste

## Preparation:

1. Preheat oven to 375°F (190°C).
2. In a large bowl, combine ground turkey, spinach, breadcrumbs (if using), egg, oregano, garlic powder, onion powder, salt, and pepper.
3. Form mixture into meatballs and place on a baking sheet.

4. Bake for 20-25 minutes, or until meatballs are cooked through.

# DAY 21: Roasted Vegetable and Quinoa Bowl

**Ingredients:**

1. 1 cup cooked quinoa
2. 1 red bell pepper, diced
3. 1 zucchini, diced
4. 1 cup cherry tomatoes, halved
5. 1 tablespoon olive oil
6. 1 teaspoon dried basil
7. Salt and pepper to taste

**Preparation:**

1. Preheat oven to 400°F (200°C).
2. Toss bell pepper, zucchini, and cherry tomatoes with olive oil, basil, salt, and pepper. Spread on a baking sheet.
3. Roast for 20-25 minutes, until vegetables are tender.

# Author's appreciation

As we conclude this meal plan, I want to extend my heartfelt appreciation for your commitment to improving your heart health through this cookbook, *Quick and Easy Low-Fat, Low-Sodium Recipes to Lower Blood Pressure, Reduce Cholesterol, and Promote Cardiovascular Health.* Your dedication to making heart-healthy choices is truly commendable and vital for maintaining your overall well-being.

This collection of recipes was carefully crafted to provide you with delicious and nutritious options that align with your health goals. Each meal is designed not only to be heart-friendly but also to bring joy to your dining experience. I hope these recipes inspire you to explore new flavors, embrace wholesome ingredients, and make heart-healthy eating a part of your everyday life.

Thank you for allowing me to be a part of your journey toward better heart health.